VAMPIRE FACIAL FOR BEGINNERS

Comprehensive Guide To Treatments, Benefits, Risks, And Techniques For Rejuvenation And Youthful Skin

DR SAWYER DIEGO

DISCLAMER

Nothing in this book should be interpreted as medical advice; it is meant exclusively for educational reasons. Regarding their specific health issues and treatment options, readers are urged to speak with licensed healthcare professionals. The publisher and author disclaim all liability for any errors or omissions in the material provided, as well as for any negative effects that may arise from using or abusing the information. Although every attempt has been taken to guarantee that the material in this book is correct as of the date of publishing, new research may have superseded some of the content because medical knowledge is always changing. It is recommended that readers confirm the most recent medical recommendations and guidelines. The reader of this book undertakes to release the author and publisher from any claims or liabilities resulting from the use of this information, and understands and accepts the inherent risks connected with healthcare decisions.

TABLE OF CONTENTS

ABOUT THE BOOK

The "Vampire Facial for Beginners" book is a must-have resource for anyone interested in learning more about this cutting-edge skincare technique. The Vampire Facial, which combines microneedling and Platelet-Rich Plasma (PRP) therapy to renew and improve skin look, was inspired by advances in cosmetic dermatology. Gaining an understanding of the procedure's definition and history is essential as it traces its development and the scientific concepts that support its efficacy.

Examining the science underlying the vampire facial clears up myths and sets it apart from other facial procedures.

This information emphasizes the vital significance of choosing a qualified provider and gives readers the ability to make educated judgments. The book guarantees treatment efficacy and safety by providing thorough instructions on examining qualifications and facility accreditation.

Before receiving a Vampire Facial, preparation is essential, and the book carefully describes skincare routines to follow as well as mental preparation strategies. It discusses possible hazards and adverse effects and provides information on how to manage discomfort and comprehend the healing process that occurs after treatment. What to expect throughout the session, including alternatives for pain control and the function of PRP in skin renewal, is made clear by the step-by-step explanation of the treatment.

To maximize recuperation, comprehensive post-treatment care instructions are provided, with an emphasis on long-term skincare advice and controlling anticipated outcomes. Benefits like enhanced skin texture, collagen stimulation, and wrinkle reduction are emphasized, along with frequently asked questions about treatment frequency and safety for a range of skin types.

Transparency and accessibility are ensured by investigating financial concerns, such as funding possibilities and average costs.

The book also covers the integration of supplementary skincare products for maintenance and compares alternatives like microneedling. By addressing frequent questions and offering thorough answers, the author makes sure that readers are equipped to handle every turn of their vampire facial experience, which inspires confidence in reaching skincare objectives.

CHAPTER ONE
VAMPIRE FACIAL OVERVIEW
UNDERSTANDING VAMPIRE FACIAL

PRP (Platelet-Rich Plasma) therapy, sometimes referred to as a vampire facial, is a cosmetic procedure that aims to renew the skin and enhance its young appearance. Due to its all-natural method of boosting skin tone, decreasing wrinkles, and improving overall texture, this therapy has become more and more popular.

The process involves extracting platelet-rich plasma, which is rich in growth factors, from the patient's blood. The creation of collagen and tissue regeneration—two processes critical to preserving youthful skin—depend on these growth factors.

A tiny amount of blood is taken from the patient's arm during a vampire facial, much like with a standard blood test. After that, the platelet-rich plasma is separated from other components of the blood using a centrifuge. After being separated, the concentrated plasma is injected directly into the desired areas of the face or administered by microneedling. Microneedling promotes the formation of collagen and increases skin suppleness by assisting in the absorption of plasma into the skin's deeper layers. The entire process involves little to no downtime, is minimally invasive, and is usually well tolerated.

A vampire facial's outcomes can change according to each person's unique skin type and issues. Nonetheless, a lot of patients report smoother, more luminous skin, and a decrease in wrinkles and fine lines.

If you want results that look natural without using harsh chemicals or unnatural fillers, this treatment is for you. All things considered, a vampire facial is a non-surgical method of skin rejuvenation that uses the body's healing abilities to support younger-looking, healthier skin.

ADVANTAGES OF A VAMPIRE FACELIFT

The advantages of a vampire facial go beyond the skin's obvious aesthetic enhancements. Its capacity to promote collagen synthesis, which is essential for preserving skin suppleness and firmness, is one of its main benefits.

As we age, the body's natural supply of collagen, a protein that supports healthy skin structure, decreases and wrinkles appear. Through a Vampire Facial, platelet-rich plasma is injected into the skin, stimulating collagen formation and eventually leading to tighter, smoother skin.

The elimination of wrinkles and fine lines is a major bonus. Platelet-rich plasma contains growth factors that aid in the restoration of injured skin cells and stimulate the development of new, healthy tissue. This procedure gives the skin a more youthful appearance by preventing the creation of new wrinkles in addition to smoothing out existing ones.

Furthermore, the process helps lessen the appearance of sun damage, hyperpigmentation, and scars by improving skin tone and texture.

A vampire facial is also safe and minimally intrusive, so it may be done on a variety of skin types and age groups. A vampire facial usually involves minimal recovery time, in contrast to regular facelift operations or chemical peels, which can include significant downtime and associated hazards. With just slight redness or swelling as possible short-term side effects, patients can return to their regular activities soon after the treatment. All things considered, the advantages of a vampire facial make it a desirable choice for people looking for long-lasting, all-natural skin regeneration.

FOR WHOM IS A VAMPIRE FACIAL BENEFICIAL?

Those who want to enhance their skin's general appearance and texture without having intrusive treatments done can benefit from a vampire facial.

It is especially helpful for people who are worried about aging symptoms like wrinkles, fine lines, and decreased skin suppleness. Sun damage, uneven skin tone, dull complexion, and acne scars can all be improved by the procedure.

A vampire facial can assist younger persons in their 20s and 30s to avoid early aging by keeping their skin looking young and delaying the appearance of fine lines and wrinkles.

 This operation can also be very beneficial to older adults who are already exhibiting signs of aging, since it helps to tighten and revitalize drooping skin, giving the illusion of younger skin.

Furthermore, people who have particular skin issues, such as hyperpigmentation or acne scars, could discover that a vampire facial improves skin texture and lessens the visibility of imperfections. Since the treatment makes use of the body's inherent healing processes, most skin types, including sensitive skin, can take it well.

Overall, a vampire facial is a good and non-invasive option for anyone hoping to have firmer, smoother, and more radiant skin without using harsh chemicals or artificial fillers.

A SYNOPSIS OF THE VAMPIRE COSMETIC PROCEDURE

A consultation with a competent practitioner who will evaluate the patient's skin issues and goals precedes the Vampire Facial procedure. A tiny amount of blood is taken from the patient's arm during the actual procedure, just like in a standard blood test.

After that, the blood is put into a centrifuge, which spins quickly to separate the platelet-rich plasma (PRP) from the other components of the blood.

Following its isolation, PRP is either injected directly onto the face or coupled with microneedling. Using a tool with small needles to make microscopic punctures on the skin's surface is known as microneedling.

Because of these microchannels, PRP can enter the skin's deeper layers, promoting the formation of collagen and accelerating the body's natural healing process.

The full vampire facial technique just takes a few hours, usually between thirty and sixty minutes. Patients may feel some slight discomfort during the injection or microneedling procedure, although pain is usually reduced by applying numbing lotion beforehand.

Similar to moderate sunburn, the skin may appear somewhat reddish or puffy after the treatment; however, these side effects normally go away in a few hours to a day.

Patients usually see modest improvements in texture, firmness, and overall complexion over the next few weeks. For best results, it would be advised to schedule numerous sessions, separated by a few weeks.

Personalized skin conditions and lifestyle variables can affect how long results stay, but with good skincare maintenance, many patients report advantages that continue for many months or even more than a year.

CHAPTER TWO
RECOGNIZING THE VAMPIRE FACE
MEANING AND HISTORY

In recent years, the Vampire Facial—also referred to as Platelet-Rich Plasma (PRP) Therapy—has grown in popularity as a revitalizing facial procedure. During this process, platelet-rich plasma is extracted from the patient's blood and subsequently put back into the skin following microneedling. The purpose of this facial is to increase the production of collagen and enhance the flexibility, tone, and texture of the skin. PRP therapy was first created to help with tissue repair and recovery in orthopedic surgery and sports medicine. Later, it was modified for cosmetic uses, especially in the area of facial aesthetics.

The history of platelet-rich plasma (PRP) therapy dates back to the use of this substance in medicine to hasten tissue recovery after injury. The idea is to apply concentrated platelets, which are high in growth factors, to areas that need rejuvenation to maximize the body's inherent healing abilities. A precise procedure is required for the facial adaptation: the patient's blood is extracted, PRP is extracted, and the blood is then strategically placed on the face. With continued use, this technique hopes to increase the skin's capacity for regeneration and a more youthful appearance.

Knowing the history of the vampire facial highlights both its medical beginnings and its entry into the cosmetic sphere, highlighting its foundation in the scientific understanding of tissue regeneration and wound healing. People can understand how the treatment evolved and how it is used in cosmetic dermatology now by learning about its history.

THE PROCEDURE'S SCIENTIFIC BASIS

The qualities of platelet-rich plasma (PRP) and its impact on skin renewal are the science behind the vampire facial. Platelets are naturally occurring components of blood that are essential for wound healing and clotting.

PRP has a high concentration of these components. Growth factors found in these platelets promote cellular regeneration and repair when administered to aging or injured skin.

A tiny sample of the patient's blood is extracted during the vampire facial surgery, and it is spun in a centrifuge to separate the plasma—which is high in platelets—from other blood components. Subsequently, the face is treated with this concentrated PRP via topical application or microneedling. Through the formation of microscopic channels in the skin's surface, PRP can thoroughly penetrate the skin and promote the development of collagen. Collagen plays a major role in decreasing wrinkles and enhancing the overall texture of skin because it is necessary for preserving the suppleness and firmness of the skin.

According to science, the Vampire Facial encourages skin renewal by utilizing the body's healing processes. Over time, the technique produces smoother, firmer skin by directly stimulating the production of new tissue and repairing damaged skin with a concentrated dose of growth factors. Knowing this procedure's scientific foundation demystifies it and emphasizes its potential advantages for anyone looking for non-surgical face rejuvenation choices.

COMMON MISCONCEPTIONS DISPELLED

The Vampire Facial is becoming more and more well-known, but certain myths about it may discourage prospective patients from getting the procedure. A frequent misperception is that the treatment entails administering blood directly into the face, which can be frightening. In actuality, the Vampire Facial employs a sophisticated procedure in which PRP—which is made from the patient's blood—is administered topically or by microneedling following meticulous processing.

There is also a myth that the Vampire's face hurts or takes a long time to recover from. With the application of numbing creams, most patients handle microneedling procedures successfully, despite the possibility of mild discomfort. The downtime after treatment is normally quite short; after a few days, there may be some redness and moderate swelling, but these side effects usually go away.

There's also a myth that the Vampire Facial produces immediate effects on par with surgery. In actuality, while collagen formation is stimulated and patients may notice changes in skin tone and texture over the coming weeks, best outcomes frequently call for numerous treatments spaced several weeks apart.

Dispelling these myths is essential for anyone thinking about getting a vampire facial since it makes the procedure's safety, method, and results more clear.

COMPARATIVE ANALYSIS OF OTHER FACE TREATMENTS

Knowing how the Vampire face stacks up against other face rejuvenation procedures can help people select the best course of action for their skincare objectives.

The Vampire Facial targets deeper skin layers to stimulate collagen formation and promote long-term skin renewal, in contrast to traditional facials that largely focus on washing and moisturizing the skin's surface.

By adding volume to specific facial areas, injectable fillers, such as hyaluronic acid, eliminate wrinkles and improve contours; in contrast, the Vampire Facial offers a more comprehensive approach to improving skin elasticity and texture overall. While injectables yield results right away, the Vampire Facial's effects take several weeks to manifest while the collagen rebuilds, providing a more natural boost.

Unlike laser treatments that target specific skin issues like acne scars or pigmentation with concentrated light energy, the Vampire Facial uses PRP therapy to stimulate the body's natural healing processes. This makes it a good choice for people searching for a low-risk, non-invasive surgery with little recovery time and results that seem natural.

Knowing these comparisons enables people to assess the advantages and factors to take into account for each face rejuvenation technique according to their tastes, needs for skincare, and intended results. Making an educated choice improves pleasure with the selected skincare regimen, whether you decide to go with the Vampire Facial for its collagen-boosting benefits or choose something else.

SELECTING A QUALIFIED PROVIDER IS CRUCIAL

It's crucial to choose a certified Vampire Facial therapist to guarantee patient safety, the best outcomes, and a satisfying experience all along the way. A skilled practitioner should be well-versed in dermatology or cosmetic medicine, with a focus on PRP therapy and facial aesthetics.

demonstrate their knowledge and dedication to patient care, they have to get licenses and certifications from respectable medical boards or associations.

Prospective patients should investigate possible providers before getting the Vampire Facial. They should look through their backgrounds, patient endorsements, and before-and-after pictures of prior procedures. People can talk about their expectations, skincare objectives, and any worries they may have regarding the process by consulting with the practitioner.

To establish whether a patient is a candidate for the Vampire Facial, a trained healthcare professional will thoroughly evaluate the patient's medical history and state of skin health. To ensure informed consent, they will go over the entire process with you, including any potential risks and advantages. They will also tailor the treatment program to each patient's unique needs to address particular skin issues and maximize outcomes.

Patients can have confidence in the safety and effectiveness of their Vampire Facial experience by selecting a qualified therapist.

CHAPTER THREE

HOW TO GET READY FOR A VAMPIRE FACIAL

FIRST ENCOUNTER WITH A PROVIDER

Set up an initial consultation with a certified practitioner before beginning your vampire facial quest. You can talk about your expectations for the procedure, your fears, and your goals during this crucial session. Your skin type, medical history, and therapy suitability will all be evaluated by the healthcare professional. They will go through the entire procedure with you, including what to anticipate both before and after the facial. You should also use this opportunity to ask any questions you may have regarding the operation, its advantages, and possible results.

The therapist will discuss how to tailor the treatment plan to meet your unique needs throughout the appointment. For best effects, they might suggest extra skincare items or procedures to go along with the vampire facial. To make sure the process is safe and successful for you, you must be open about any allergies, prescription drugs, or skin issues you may have. The consultation ensures that you are comfortable and well-informed before the vampire facial, and it also sets the stage for a collaborative approach between you and your physician.

PRE-OPERATIVE SKIN CARE PROTOCOL

A customized skincare routine is necessary to prime your skin for a vampire facial to maximize benefits and reduce risks. Your doctor will give you pre-operation skin care instructions, which can include moisturizing, exfoliating, and maybe avoiding certain products like retinoids or exfoliants for a few days before to the procedure. The goal of this routine is to make sure your skin is in the best possible condition and prepared to absorb the advantages of the facial.

During this preparatory stage, it's important to stay hydrated and shield your skin from the sun and other damaging environmental factors.

To maximize the revitalizing benefits of the vampire facial, your therapist could suggest using particular serums or creams on the days before your session. Paying close attention to these recommendations promotes the general health of your skin and aids in creating a smooth canvas for the operation.

POSSIBLE DANGERS AND ADVERSE REACTIONS

Comprehending the possible hazards and adverse reactions associated with a vampire facial is vital for making well-informed choices.

Temporary redness, swelling, or moderate soreness at the injection sites are common side effects, however, these are usually regarded harmless when administered by a qualified physician. Some people might get bruises, particularly if they have delicate skin or are prone to getting bruises easily.

Infection, allergic responses to treatment ingredients, and uneven skin texture are less frequent hazards.

During your consultation, your provider will go over these risks with you and provide you with tips on how to reduce them. Adherence to post-procedure care instructions is essential to minimize problems and facilitate healing. You can approach the operation with reasonable expectations and faith in your provider's experience if you are informed of these possible consequences.

TIPS FOR BOTH MENTAL AND PHYSICAL READYING

To guarantee a great experience and the best possible outcomes, there are a few practical things to do to psychologically and physically prepare for a vampire facial.

First, in the days before your appointment, it's beneficial to keep hydrated and eat a balanced diet. Sufficient moisture facilitates the processes of skin renewal and repair. Better skin health and general well-being can also be attributed to obtaining enough sleep and controlling stress levels.

It's common to experience some mental trepidation or fear before any cosmetic operation. Deep breathing exercises and meditation are examples of relaxation practices that can help reduce anxiety and foster optimism. Imagining the result you want from your vampire facial can also inspire excitement and confidence. To clear up any doubts you may have, don't forget to discuss any worries or inquiries you may have with your provider at the appointment.

FAQS: WHAT SHOULD I STAY AWAY FROM BEFORE THE PROCEDURE?

It's best to stay away from specific skincare products and treatments in the days leading up to your vampire facial since they may cause issues or exacerbate sensitivity. This entails staying away from chemical peels, abrasive exfoliants, and prolonged sun exposure. These goods and practices have the potential to aggravate skin conditions or increase their likelihood, such as redness or inflammation, both during and after facial procedures.

Additionally, since retinoids and vitamin A derivatives can make skin more sensitive, it is advised to avoid using them the week before your treatment. Likewise, limiting the use of vitamins or drugs that thin the blood, such as fish oil or aspirin, can lessen the chance of bruises at the injection sites. To guarantee you get the most out of your vampire facial, your therapist will provide you with customized instructions based on your skin type and medical background.

CHAPTER FOUR

AN EXPLANATION OF THE VAMPIRE FACIAL PROCEDURE

DETAILED PROCEDURE

PRP (Platelet-Rich Plasma) therapy, commonly referred to as the "Vampire Facial," is a series of essential procedures designed to revitalize the skin and give it a more youthful appearance. Initially, the physician will take a tiny sample of blood from your arm, much like they would during a standard blood test. After that, the platelets—which contain growth factors with regeneration potential—are separated from the blood in a centrifuge. To enhance comfort during the process, the skin is numbed with a topical anesthetic once the PRP is prepared.

Next, a microneedling tool is used to delicately apply PRP to the face, or the substance is injected directly into the areas that require therapy. Because microneedling makes microscopic channels in the skin's surface, PRP can enter the skin deeply and promote the production of collagen. This increase in collagen helps to improve the general tone and flexibility of the skin, minimize wrinkles and fine lines, and improve skin texture. Any leftover PRP may be rubbed into the skin for optimal absorption following the PRP treatment.

It usually takes between sixty and ninety minutes to complete the process, depending on the areas that need to be treated and the particular method your practitioner uses. Following that, you might have some moderate swelling or redness, but these symptoms normally go away in a few hours to a day. As collagen continues to rebuild over several weeks, the results steadily get better, giving you smoother, younger-looking skin.

AN OVERVIEW OF THE EQUIPMENT USED

The main pieces of equipment needed for a vampire facial operation are a centrifuge, a microneedling tool, and many sterile medical supplies. By rapidly spinning the blood, the centrifuge is essential for isolating the platelet-rich plasma (PRP) from the other components of the blood. The platelets are separated during this process and subsequently gathered for topical application. When used in conjunction with PRP, the microneedling device's tiny needles induce controlled micro-injuries in the skin, which encourage the creation of collagen and elastin.

To ensure patient comfort during the operation, additional necessary equipment includes topical numbing creams or gels and sterile syringes for injecting PRP and taking blood.

To reduce the danger of infection and guarantee the best possible outcomes, all equipment is meticulously sanitized and maintained by medical standards. Each piece of equipment required to give safe and effective PRP therapy customized to your skin's needs will be explained by your practitioner.

RECOGNIZING PLATELET-RICH PLASMA (PRP)

Platelet-rich plasma, or PRP, is a concentrated serum made from your blood that is rich in growth factors, other bioactive proteins, and platelets. When administered to the skin during a vampire facial, these platelets are essential for tissue regeneration, healing, and restoration.

A tiny amount of the patient's blood is extracted, and the plasma and platelets are separated from the red blood cells using a centrifuge to produce platelet-rich plasma (PRP).

The resultant platelet-derived growth factor (PRP) is abundant in growth factors, including VEGF (vascular endothelial growth factor), TGF-beta (transforming growth factor), and PDGF (platelet-derived growth factor), which promote collagen synthesis and cell renewal. PRP improves overall skin tone, minimizes wrinkles, and improves skin texture when injected or administered topically.

Because the patient's blood is used, there is a lower chance of allergic reactions or rejection, making it a safe and natural therapy choice.

PRP therapy is becoming more and more popular for treating joint pain, hair loss, and sports injuries in addition to cosmetic rejuvenation. Because of its regenerative qualities, patients can benefit from a variety of therapy options that are supported by clinical trials and scientific research, resulting in little downtime and excellent outcomes.

OPTIONS FOR PAIN MANAGEMENT

Topical anesthetic creams or gels are usually given to the skin before the start of the Vampire Facial procedure to manage pain. These anesthetics aid in reducing any pain brought on by PRP injections or the microneedling procedure.

To provide the patient with a comfortable experience, the numbing cream is typically applied 30 to 45 minutes before to the treatment.

To reduce their discomfort even more during microneedling or PRP injections, patients may choose to use extra painkillers like ice packs or cold air devices. Before the process, your practitioner will go over these alternatives with you to address any concerns and make sure you're comfortable during the treatment session.

To ensure that the experience meets your needs, it's critical to be transparent with your healthcare practitioner about your preferences for pain management and your level of pain tolerance.

During the vampire facial process, practitioners can improve patient relaxation and overall experience by utilizing efficient pain control measures.

This method maximizes the benefits of PRP therapy for skin regeneration and renewal while ensuring patients may comfortably undergo treatment.

FAQS: WHAT IS THE DURATION OF THE PROCEDURE?

A vampire facial usually takes between sixty and ninety minutes to complete, depending on several variables, such as the areas treated and the particular method your practitioner uses. First, a small amount of blood is drawn from your arm and processed in a centrifuge to separate the platelet-rich plasma (PRP). Typically, this preparatory process takes fifteen to twenty minutes.

After the PRP is prepared, a topical anesthetic is applied to the skin to numb it; this process takes an extra 30 to 45 minutes to take full effect.

Using injections or microneedling, the actual PRP application takes 20 to 30 minutes, depending on the complexity and degree of treatment required. Following the procedure, further time could be needed to take care of any urgent post-treatment care needs or to massage any leftover PRP into the skin.

Vampire Facial is intended to be a rather simple and quick outpatient procedure that works well with most schedules. After treatment, patients can usually resume their regular activities right once, though there may be some mild redness or swelling that goes away in a day or two. The following weeks are typically when the procedure's best effects become apparent as collagen creation keeps enhancing the texture and look of the skin.

CHAPTER FIVE

RECUPERATION AND AFTERCARE

QUICK AFTERCARE GUIDELINES

It's essential to adhere to the aftercare guidelines right away following a vampire facial to promote the best possible recovery and outcomes. Your skin may feel sensitive and seem somewhat red, similar to a little sunburn, just after the surgery. To avoid irritating your face, try not to touch or rub it too much. A calming serum or moisturizer may be applied by your skincare expert to help the skin relax and heal more quickly.

Unless otherwise directed, refrain from washing your face or using any makeup for the first few hours. It's common to feel a little tight or uncomfortable, but you may calm the skin and reduce swelling by gently applying cold packs wrapped in a soft towel. To help drain out toxins and encourage skin hydration from the inside out, stay hydrated by drinking lots of water.

Avoid direct sunlight and heat exposure even after the first redness goes down over the next few hours. If you must go outside, protect your skin by donning a broad-spectrum sunscreen with SPF 30 or greater. To guarantee optimal outcomes and thorough healing of your skin, adhere to any post-treatment advice given by your skincare specialist.

HANDLING PAIN AND SWELLING

Controlling soreness and edema following a vampire facial is crucial for smooth recuperation. It is typical and expected for you to feel somewhat swollen and tender right after the treatment. Apply cold compresses or ice packs covered in a cloth to the affected areas for ten to fifteen minutes at a time to reduce discomfort. This relieves any discomfort and lessens edema.

For the first twenty-four hours, stay away from intense exercise and hard face motions to avoid aggravating edema. Reducing fluid retention in the facial tissues might also be aided by slightly elevating your head when you're lying down. If you are in any discomfort, your skincare professional might suggest over-the-counter pain medicines like acetaminophen; however, stay away from aspirin and ibuprofen as they may cause bruising.

Stick to mild skincare regimens and refrain from using abrasive products or exfoliants that can irritate your skin during the first stages of recuperation. To promote ideal healing and reduce swelling, adhere to any special post-procedure advice given by your skincare specialist. See your provider for more advice if the swelling continues or becomes noticeably severe.

TIMELINE FOR EXPECTED OUTCOMES

It's possible to successfully manage expectations and track progress by being aware of the timeframe for expected results following a vampire facial. As the therapy begins to take action, you might see some initial improvements in skin tone and texture in the first 24-48 hours after the operation.

Mild redness and swelling, however, are commonplace during this initial phase and usually go away in one to three days.

The facial stimulates the creation of collagen, which gradually improves the suppleness and firmness of the skin over the next few weeks. Within 1-2 weeks of treatment, many people report observable improvements in skin texture, smaller pores, and a more radiant complexion. Over the following three to six months, when the processes of collagen remodeling and regeneration take place, the results get better.

Adhere to a consistent skincare routine suited to your skin type and issues to maximize and sustain benefits. As advised by your skincare professional, schedule follow-up consultations to evaluate your progress and modify your treatment plan as needed. You can get long-lasting results from your vampire facial by following post-procedure care instructions and adopting healthy skincare practices.

LONG-TERM ADVICE FOR SKIN CARE

Developing long-term skincare routines can help maintain effects and enhance general skin health following a vampire facial. To protect your skin from UV damage, incorporate a daily skincare routine that includes moisturizers, broad-spectrum sunscreen with SPF 30 or higher, and mild cleansers. When you're outside, shield yourself from the sun by wearing clothing and accessories.

To encourage the formation of collagen and preserve skin hydration, think about using serums or creams that include hyaluronic acid, vitamins C and E, or peptides. Frequent exfoliation can improve product absorption by removing dead skin cells with moderate scrapes or chemical exfoliants. Hydrate your skin from the inside out by consuming enough water each day and eating a well-balanced diet full of vital minerals and antioxidants.

For individualized advice and treatments, speak with your skin care specialist if you've seen any changes in your skin or have specific concerns. Make routine follow-up consultations to track skin improvement and make any adjustments to your skincare routine. You can extend the effects of your vampire facial and attain long-lasting skin rejuvenation by investing in proactive and persistent skincare routines.

FAQS: AFTER THE SURGERY, WHAT SHOULD I NOT DO?

You must abstain from activities that can impair the healing process and outcomes of your vampire facial. Avoid strenuous exercise, heavy lifting, and activities that cause excessive perspiration during the first 24 to 48 hours. Engaging in these activities may worsen swelling or bruises by increasing blood flow to the face.

To avoid skin irritation and hyperpigmentation during the early phase of recuperation, stay out of the sun and avoid being in the heat. If you must go outside, shield your skin from UV radiation by donning a wide-brimmed hat and using a broad-spectrum sunscreen with an SPF of 30 or higher. Reducing alcohol intake and smoking can help improve skin repair and collagen production.

For at least a week following the procedure, use caution when using skincare products and treatments that could irritate your skin, such as retinoids, chemical peels, or harsh exfoliants. If your skincare specialist gives you particular aftercare recommendations, follow them to maximize healing and reduce the chance of problems. For advice and assistance, get in touch with your provider if you have questions or notice strange symptoms.

CHAPTER SIX

ADVANTAGES OF A VAMPIRE FACELIFT

COLLAGEN BOOSTING AND SKIN REJUVENATION

A vampire facial is a popular option for people who want youthful, glowing skin since it provides substantial benefits for collagen stimulation and skin renewal. The face is thoroughly cleansed before the operation to get rid of any oils, debris, or makeup. To ensure patient comfort throughout the procedure, a topical numbing lotion is then given. Taking a small sample of the patient's blood, usually from the arm, is the essential part of the vampire facial. The platelet-rich plasma (PRP) is then separated using a centrifuge.

When injected into the face or administered topically following microneedling, PRP's abundance of growth factors promotes the formation of collagen and cell regeneration.

By making microscopic punctures in the skin's surface, microneedling promotes the skin's natural healing process and enhances PRP absorption. Over time, this mixture encourages skin that is smoother, tighter and has better elasticity and texture.

The Vampire Facial has slow but significant benefits; many patients see an increase in collagen synthesis and refined skin texture within a few weeks, giving them a more youthful appearance. For people who want to fight aging symptoms and get a young glow, the Vampire Facial is a great alternative because regular sessions can further improve these benefits.

ENHANCING TONE AND TEXTURE OF SKIN

Improving skin tone and texture by treating problems like roughness, uneven pigmentation, and acne scars is one of the main advantages of the vampire facial. To preserve the structure and suppleness of the skin, new collagen and elastin fibers must be produced, and this is accomplished in part by the microneedling procedure. Because PRP is high in growth factors, it accelerates the rejuvenation and cell turnover processes, which amplifies these effects.

During the procedure, the skin is deliberately micro-injured by the microneedling device, which stimulates the skin to produce new collagen and elastin in an attempt to mend itself. This procedure helps to reduce the visibility of pores and fine wrinkles in addition to improving the skin's general texture. PRP therapy helps the skin absorb more healthy nutrients and speeds up healing, giving the complexion a smoother, more even tone.

Following a vampire facial, patients usually experience incremental changes in skin tone and texture over a few weeks; the best benefits usually show after numerous sessions.

REDUCING WRINKLES AND FINE LINES

Due to its collagen-boosting qualities and skin-rejuvenating effects, the vampire facial is frequently used to treat fine lines and wrinkles.

As we age, fine lines and wrinkles appear because our skin naturally loses collagen and elastin. The Vampire Facial fights this by using PRP therapy and microneedling to increase the production of collagen.

The skin's natural healing reaction is triggered during the process by the microscopic punctures made on the skin's surface by the microneedling device. As a result, new collagen and elastin fibers are produced, firming and plumping the skin and gradually lessening the visibility of wrinkles and fine lines. By supplying growth factors to the skin directly, PRP therapy accelerates these effects and promotes faster cell turnover and regeneration.

Following a course of Vampire Facial treatments, many patients report smoother, more youthful-looking skin, with improvements in fine lines and wrinkles becoming more noticeable with each session. Due to its non-invasive nature and little recovery time, the procedure is a great choice for people who lead busy lives and want the benefits of anti-aging without having to deal with the lengthy recovery period that comes with more invasive treatments.

TAKING CARE OF HYPERPIGMENTATION

A Vampire Facial's mix of microneedling and PRP therapy makes it an excellent treatment for hyperpigmentation, which is characterized by dark spots or patches on the skin. PRP provides growth factors that encourage uniform skin tone and lessen discoloration, while microneedling aids in the disruption of pigment clusters and encourages the creation of new, healthy skin cells.

The PRP can fully penetrate the skin and target areas of hyperpigmentation since the microneedling equipment forms microscopic channels in the skin during the treatment. Through this process, the skin is encouraged to replace damaged pigmented cells with new, equally toned skin. Patients usually see a more even complexion and a decrease in the appearance of dark patches with time.

Sunspots, age spots, and post-inflammatory hyperpigmentation are among the hyperpigmentation that can be treated with the vampire facial. The skin continues to renew and rejuvenate over several weeks, resulting in slow but noticeable improvements.

FAQ: HOW FREQUENTLY IS A VAMPIRE FACIAL POSSIBLE?

Regarding the Vampire Facial, one of the most often queries is how many sessions are required to get and keep the best results. Skin tone, texture, and fine wrinkles can initially be improved by beginning with a series of three treatments spaced approximately four to six weeks apart, according to dermatologist recommendations. Depending on the specific skin issues and objectives of each patient, maintenance treatments are usually advised six months to a year following this initial series.

The period between treatments maximizes the benefits of collagen stimulation and cell renewal while giving the skin ample time to repair and regenerate. For those with more serious skin issues, more sessions can be helpful, while for others, maintenance treatments every six months might be enough to keep the desired effects.

It's crucial to speak with a licensed dermatologist or skincare specialist to figure out the best course of action for your skin type, issues, and goals. They can evaluate how your skin has responded to the vampire facial and create a customized timetable that will optimize the benefits while maintaining the long-term health and integrity of your skin.

CHAPTER SEVEN

POSSIBLE DANGERS AND ADVERSE REACTIONS

TYPICAL ADVERSE EFFECTS AND THEIR MANAGEMENT

Mild side effects like redness, edema, and sensitivity in the treated area are typical following a vampire facial. These symptoms can be controlled with easy steps, and they usually go away in a few hours to a day. Reducing swelling and relieving any discomfort can be achieved by applying cold packs or ice wrapped in a cloth.

Additionally, redness can be reduced and skin can be kept hydrated by utilizing gentle skincare products like moisturizers or calming creams that have been advised by your physician.

Though rare, more serious side effects could include mild skin irritation or bruises. If there is any bruising, it normally goes away in a week. To reduce the possibility of aggravating these adverse effects, stay out of the sun and avoid physically demanding activities during the first 24 hours after starting treatment. It's advisable to get in touch with your skincare provider if you notice severe or persistent responses that go beyond what is considered normal to ensure appropriate evaluation and advice on how to proceed with therapy.

Your vampire facial will be more successful overall and your recuperation process will go more smoothly if you are aware of the typical side effects and know how to handle them. You can minimize any short-term discomfort while maximizing the advantages of your treatment and promoting healing by adhering to these useful suggestions.

RISKS OF INFECTION AND ALLERGIC REACTIONS

Although infections and allergic reactions are uncommon with vampire facials, it's important to be aware of the dangers to receive safe treatment. In the treated region, allergic responses may cause hives, rashes, or itching. To reduce these risks, you must let your provider know about any known allergies or sensitivities before the treatment. To evaluate possible side effects and confirm that the treatment is appropriate for your skin type, providers frequently do a patch test in advance.

By maintaining stringent hygiene during the operation, infection risks are reduced. Throughout, your provider should keep everything tidy and utilize sterile equipment.

Typically, aftercare guidelines ask for keeping the treated area dry and clean and avoiding excessive contact with it. You must get in touch with your provider right away if you observe any infection-related symptoms, such as increased redness, swelling, or warmth associated with pus or fever. Timely medical intervention can avert problems and guarantee appropriate therapy.

Knowing the potential for allergic reactions and infections gives you the ability to protect your skin's health both before and after a vampire facial. You may reduce these dangers and safely reap the rewards of smoother, more youthful skin by following your skin care professional's pre-procedure and post-care instructions.

COMPREHENDING THE HEALING PROCESS

After a vampire facial, various phases in the healing process affect the treatment's overall outcome. You might have some moderate swelling and redness right after the surgery; these are natural side effects that usually go away in a day or two.

Your skin begins to rejuvenate and mend during this period, propelled by the growth hormones and nutrients administered during the facial.

As collagen production rises over the next few days to weeks, you may notice improvements in the texture, tone, and suppleness of your skin. To aid in the healing process, you must adhere to your provider's recommendations about skincare practices and sun protection. Results can be improved and skin health maintained by using moisturizers and mild cleansers that are advised for post-facial care.

Because individual results may vary depending on skin type and the specific conditions treated, patience is essential during the healing process. Having follow-up meetings with your provider enables you to evaluate your progress and make any necessary changes to your skincare regimen. Comprehending the stages of recuperation aids in controlling anticipations and guarantees the best possible results from your vampire facial.

WHEN TO GET IN TOUCH WITH YOUR SUPPLIER

After a vampire facial, knowing when to get in touch with your provider can guarantee that you get quick advice and assistance as you heal. While certain signs of moderate redness, swelling, or bruises are typical, others need to be treated right away. You must get in touch with your skincare specialist right away if you encounter severe discomfort, persistent swelling, or infection symptoms like pus, warmth, or fever.

Additionally, consulting a physician guarantees appropriate intervention if you observe unexpected changes in skin texture or pigmentation, or if the treated region does not appear to be healing as predicted.

To maximize outcomes, your provider may recommend extra treatments or changes to your skincare routine in addition to recommendations catered to your particular needs.

Maintaining open lines of communication with your skincare specialist encourages working together to safely and successfully achieve your skincare objectives. You can prolong the benefits of your vampire facial and keep your skin looking young and healthy by taking care of any issues as soon as they arise.

FAQS: CAN ANYONE GET A VAMPIRE FACIAL?

Most people can safely receive vampire facials when they are done by a trained skincare specialist utilizing sterile procedures and the right guidelines. However, some people may not be able to receive this treatment due to specific issues. Vampire facials are generally not recommended for expectant or nursing mothers because of possible health hazards to the fetus or baby.

To avoid aggravating or spreading, people with active skin infections, such as cold sores or acne breakouts, should also hold off on therapy until these diseases clear up. Before getting a vampire facial, people with a history of keloid scarring or slow wound healing might need to have their skincare professional carefully evaluate them and provide individualized suggestions.

You must inform your provider of any allergies, medical conditions, or drugs you are taking during the initial consultation to ensure safety and efficacy. This enables them to determine if you are a good candidate for the therapy and customize the process to meet your specific requirements. Smoother, more radiant skin is something you can confidently enjoy by prioritizing skin health and taking professional advice.

CHAPTER EIGHT
SELECTING AN ELIGIBLE SUPPLIER
INVESTIGATING EXPERIENCE AND CREDENTIALS

It's important to look into a vampire facial provider's past in great detail while investigating their experience and credentials. Verify their training and educational background first. A trustworthy practitioner should have experience in dermatology, plastic surgery, or a similar discipline; preferably, they should have received specialized training in aesthetic procedures such as vampire facials. Seek certifications from reputable dermatological or aesthetic medicine groups or boards of medicine. This guarantees that they have fulfilled specified training and practice requirements.

Experience is just as important. Ask the practitioner how long they have been doing vampire facials and how often they do them. Expert practitioners are typically more knowledgeable about the architecture of the face and can produce outcomes that are both more effective and less problematic. Customer evaluations and reviews can also reveal information about the competence of the provider and patient happiness.

You can check internet directories of medical experts, go to the provider's website, or get in touch with local medical boards to confirm credentials. Never be afraid to question the provider directly about their background, education, and any other credentials they might possess. Finding a certified supplier that can carry out the surgery safely and successfully is ensured by a thorough research process.

FACILITY CERTIFICATION

Selecting a vampire facial provider who has certification for their establishment is essential to guaranteeing standards of quality and safety. An impartial accrediting body has rigorously reviewed the facility's procedures, supplies, and personnel credentials to grant accreditation.

This procedure guarantees that the institution satisfies or surpasses predetermined criteria for hygiene and care.

Strict guidelines for patient safety, equipment sterilization, and infection control are usually followed by accredited facilities. They also keep up with the necessary emergency processes and have plans in place for dealing with complexities, should they occur. You may be sure your vampire facial will be done in a clean, safe setting if you choose an approved facility.

The Joint Commission and the Accreditation Association for Ambulatory Health Care (AAAHC) are two examples of organizations that may grant accreditation.

These organizations assess hospitals according to certain standards, such as patient outcomes, facility administration, and patient care procedures. Selecting a facility that has received accreditation shows that it is dedicated to providing high-quality care and guarantees that you will have your vampire facial in a setting that puts your health first.

CUSTOMER TESTIMONIALS AND REVIEWS

Customer reviews and testimonials offer insightful information about what it's like for patients to visit a vampire facial provider. Spend some time reading reviews on reliable websites like Google, Yelp, or the provider's website before selecting a supplier. To obtain a fair assessment of their services, pay attention to both favorable and negative reviews.

Positive evaluations frequently emphasize features like efficient outcomes, little discomfort experienced during the process, and kind personnel. They can provide you with confidence regarding the provider's capacity to produce acceptable results. On the other hand, unfavorable reviews could highlight problems like protracted wait times, inadequate communication, or subpar outcomes. You may steer clear of such hazards and make an informed selection with the aid of these reviews.

Ask the practitioner for references or before-and-after pictures of past patients who have had vampire facials in addition to internet reviews. You can get a better understanding of the provider's abilities and the kinds of outcomes you might anticipate from this visual proof.

In the end, before deciding to undergo treatment, clients' endorsements and reviews are invaluable resources for determining the standing and dependability of a vampire facial provider.

QUESTIONS TO ASK DURING CONSULTATION

Asking the proper questions is crucial to obtaining information from your vampire face provider and making sure you feel comfortable proceeding with treatment. Begin by finding out about the credentials and experience of the practitioner, including any certificates they may have and their training in cosmetic operations. This demonstrates their training and experience in giving vampire facials.

Next, enquire as to the precise steps that comprise the vampire face treatment. Recognize the dangers and side effects of the treatment, as well as how it operates and the results you might anticipate. Provide specifics on the procedure's length, the healing period, and any advice for aftercare. This information assists you in managing your expectations for the procedure's results and being ready physically and psychologically for it.

Talk about the vampire facial's price as well as any possible extra charges for follow-up visits or aftercare items. Find out how to pay, if the provider takes medical insurance, and if they have financing options. It's important to comprehend the financial aspects to avoid surprises on the road.

Finally, enquire about the facility that will host the surgery. Make sure it has the required safety precautions and is accredited. Inquire about the physician's method of treating patients and how they handle problems or emergencies. You give yourself the power to decide whether to move forward with a vampire facial treatment by thoroughly questioning the consultation.

FAQ: WHERE CAN I GO FOR A TRUSTWORTHY SUPPLIER?

There are a few important things to take while looking for a reliable vampire facial provider to make sure you get a good, safe treatment. Start by looking up local medical professionals who practice aesthetic medicine or cosmetic dermatology. Seek out service providers who specialize in vampire facials, and make sure to review their qualifications, including their training and credentials.

Examine internet reviews and client feedback to determine patient happiness and results. While unfavorable evaluations may raise concerns about a provider's practice, positive reviews might show a provider's dependability and capacity to produce the required results. Make use of reliable review sites and ask friends and family who have received comparable treatments for recommendations.

Make a list of the questions you would like to ask the provider at the consultation regarding their background, the procedure, and what to anticipate before, during, and after treatment. Evaluate how they communicate and whether they are willing to resolve your problems. Reputable healthcare providers put the needs and safety of their patients first, give concise explanations, and set reasonable expectations for their recovery and outcomes.

Make sure the facility performing the treatment is accredited and follows stringent safety and hygienic guidelines. The hospital is guaranteed to meet or surpass industry standards for patient care and treatment outcomes by holding accreditation from reputable organizations. You may choose a reliable source for your vampire facial treatment with confidence if you do your homework and ask the right questions.

CHAPTER NINE

COST FACTORS AND AVAILABLE FINANCING

THE MEAN PRICE OF VAMPIRE FACIALS

A vampire facial's price might vary significantly based on several variables. You should budget between $800 and $1,500 per session on average. This price usually covers the treatment, any follow-up sessions, and the first consultation.

A few variables that affect the price are the clinic's location, the provider's background and standing, and the particular methods employed in the treatment. Large cities typically have higher fees for clinics than do smaller towns or rural locations. Furthermore, practitioners with a high level of recognition or expertise in cosmetic operations could charge more.

It's crucial to remember that pricing policies might vary greatly throughout clinics, so it's best to shop around and compare costs before choosing one.

Package discounts for several sessions are sometimes available at clinics, which can lower the total cost of care. But be wary of unusually low pricing, as these could be a sign of inexperienced suppliers or inferior products. When weighing costs, always give the provider's reputation and credentials top priority because your safety and satisfaction should come first.

Knowing how much a vampire facial typically costs might help you organize your finances and create a budget. You can choose where to get this surgery done with greater knowledge if you investigate nearby clinics and learn what variables affect costs.

FACTORS AFFECTING THE PRICE

The cost of vampire facials is influenced by several important aspects. The clinic's geographic location is among the most important. For cosmetic procedures like vampire facials, prices are usually higher in urban areas and higher-cost places. Additionally, these clinics could have higher overhead expenses, which show up in their fee schedules. Furthermore, the provider's experience and reputation are quite important. Well-known doctors who have a history of happy clientele and successful surgeries frequently charge extra for their services.

The particular methods employed in the Vampire Facial may also affect cost. Certain clinics may employ cutting-edge machinery or exclusive techniques to support their premium pricing points. Furthermore, the type of PRP (Platelet-Rich Plasma) preparation and other material quality can have an impact on the final cost. Clinics that spend more on top-of-the-line tools and premium supplies might bill more than those that use generic or basic items.

Last but not least, the demand for vampire facials can affect the cost. Popular procedures may cost more because there is a greater demand for them and a shortage of qualified providers. On the other hand, clinics that run seasonal specials or promotional discounts could temporarily drop their pricing to draw in new customers.

When thinking about a vampire facial, being aware of these aspects enables you to weigh the benefits and possible effects of various pricing possibilities.

CONSIDERATIONS FOR INSURANCE COVERAGE

Vampire facials are usually not covered by insurance since they are seen as cosmetic procedures. Since cosmetic procedures are optional and not medically required, most health insurance plans do not cover them, including PRP therapy, which is used in vampire facials. Generally speaking, insurance companies only pay for procedures that are judged medically required to address an accident or medical condition that has been identified.

Therefore, anyone thinking about getting a vampire facial should budget for paying for the treatment out of pocket. To make the expense more affordable, certain clinics could provide financing choices or payment schedules. You must ask questions about these possibilities when you first meet with a provider. It's also worth checking with your benefits administrator to see whether you can use pre-tax cash from some health savings accounts (HSAs) or flexible spending accounts (FSAs) to pay for cosmetic operations.

The fact that vampire facials are not covered by insurance emphasizes how crucial financial planning and budgeting are when thinking about cosmetic procedures. Without depending on insurance reimbursement, you can make well-informed judgments about your aesthetic goals by planning for out-of-pocket costs and looking into financing possibilities.

PLANS FOR PAYMENT AND AVAILABLE FINANCING

To assist customers in affording vampire facials and other cosmetic procedures, many clinics provide payment plans and financing alternatives. With payment plans, you can more easily manage the expense of treatment within your budget by spreading it out over several months. Usually, these plans call for a down payment and then monthly payments until the entire amount is paid off. Before accepting a payment plan, it's important to find out all the specifics, including interest rates and late payment penalties, as terms can differ between clinics.

Options for funding might also be offered by independent lenders who focus on financing for healthcare. These lenders provide loans with terms ranging from short-term funding to prolonged repayment periods, primarily for cosmetic and medical operations. To choose the best lender for your circumstances, check interest rates and credit requirements from several lenders.

Make sure you understand the entire cost and all associated costs by thoroughly reading the terms and circumstances before committing to a payment plan or financing option. For a limited period, certain clinics may provide promotional financing with low or 0% interest rates.

If you can pay off the balance within the promotional period, this can be a beneficial option.

By looking into financing and payment options, you can pursue cosmetic procedures like vampire facials without having to worry about breaking the bank. You can invest in your aesthetic aspirations with assurance and peace of mind if you select a plan that fits your financial objectives and budget.

FAQ: CAN VAMPIRE FACIALS BE COVERED BY INSURANCE?

Since vampire facials and other cosmetic operations are seen as elective treatments, insurance usually does not cover them. Insurance companies do not consider cosmetic procedures, such as PRP therapy used in vampire facials, to be medically required. As a result, patients should anticipate having to cover these costs out of pocket.

Insurance coverage does not usually apply to cosmetic operations; however, there can be an exemption if PRP therapy is utilized for medical reasons, such as orthopedic therapies or wound healing. In these cases, coverage would be determined by the particular diagnosis and medical indication rather than by the procedure's cosmetic nature.

To help manage the out-of-pocket costs, patients thinking about getting a vampire facial can ask about the financing alternatives and payment plans that the clinics offer. Certain clinics might give flexible financing options or take health savings accounts (HSAs) or flexible spending accounts (FSAs) as payment methods, which can offer tax benefits for medical costs.

Comprehending the constraints of insurance coverage for Vampire Facials enables patients to make appropriate plans and investigate substitute funding alternatives to accomplish their desired appearance. Patients who are financially educated about cosmetic operations can make well-informed judgments that fit their needs and goals.

CHAPTER TEN

INVESTIGATING COMPLEMENTARY AND ALTERNATIVE THERAPIES

A COMPARISON BETWEEN VAMPIRE FACIALS AND MICRO-NEEDLING

Although vampire facials and microneedling are both well-liked skin-rejuvenation procedures, their methods and advantages are very different. By making tiny punctures in the skin with fine needles, microneedling improves the texture of the skin and stimulates the formation of collagen. It works well to smooth out fine wrinkles, lessen acne scars, and even out skin tone. Both derma rollers and microneedling devices, which encourage skin renewal through controlled harm, can be used for therapy.

In contrast, Vampire Facials, sometimes called Platelet-Rich Plasma (PRP) facials, use microneedling followed by the injection or application of PRP made from the patient's blood to the skin. Growth factors found in PRP further promote the synthesis of collagen and elastin, speeding up the rejuvenation process. For individuals who want to attain a more youthful appearance, decrease hyperpigmentation, and increase skin elasticity, vampire facials are perfect.

Your unique skin issues and treatment objectives will determine which of the two procedures—microneedling or vampire facials—to use. With little downtime and a progressive improvement in a variety of skin types and diseases, microneedling is a flexible procedure.

On the other hand, vampire facials are especially advantageous for anti-aging benefits and general skin regeneration because they yield better outcomes in collagen stimulation and skin rejuvenation.

COMBINATION TREATMENTS FOR BETTER OUTCOMES

The results of vampire facials can be greatly improved by combining them with other alternative therapies.

Combining chemical peels with vampire facials is one efficient combo. Chemical peels remove dead skin cells from the skin's surface, allowing PRP to enter the skin more deeply and work its renewing magic. Combining these two benefits smoothes out the texture of the face, minimizes fine wrinkles, and treats acne scars.

Combining laser treatments with vampire facials is another advantageous combination. Fractional laser therapy and IPL (Intense Pulsed Light) are examples of laser therapies that target particular skin issues such as uneven skin tone, age spots, and sun damage. Laser treatments efficiently improve skin tone and clarity and can speed up the creation of collagen when paired with PRP from vampire facials.

In addition, interspersing microneedling treatments with vampire facials can help to preserve and improve results over time. By increasing collagen synthesis, microneedling prepares the skin for PRP therapy during later vampire facial procedures. By extending the advantages of both procedures, this synergistic strategy guarantees long-term skin renewal and an increase in the general health of the skin.

To achieve the most comprehensive skincare advantages and enhance treatment efficacy, it is recommended to combine vampire facials with other skincare therapies according to your skin's unique needs.

HOMEMADE VS. EXPERT TREATMENTS

The decision to undergo professional or DIY Vampire Facial treatments has a big impact on the efficacy and safety of the procedure. Using PRP made from own blood samples or using home microneedling equipment are common DIY techniques. Although do-it-yourself kits might seem convenient, if they are not used in a sterile environment, there is a risk of infection and incorrect technique.

Professional vampire facials guarantee correct sterilization and method adherence when performed by dermatologists or skincare specialists with training. To reduce the danger of infection and increase the effectiveness of treatment, professionals utilize sterile PRP preparation and medical-grade microneedling equipment. Professional treatments also enable the customization of PRP concentrations to meet the specific demands of each patient's skin, guaranteeing the best possible rejuvenation outcomes.

Depending on your skin type and issues, a skincare professional's experience is crucial in selecting the right treatment intensity and frequency. To safely obtain desired results, they can also monitor how your skin responds to therapy and modify procedures as necessary. Professional vampire facials provide patients with a piece of mind because they can undergo treatments in a safe setting and can seek medical advice if necessary.

DIY methods, on the other hand, do not provide the individualized evaluation and professional supervision required for safe and efficient skincare results.

INCLUDING SKINCARE ITEMS IN MAINTENANCE

Including the right skincare products in your routine is essential to maintaining the outcomes of vampire facials. Gentle cleansers, moisturizing serums, and moisturizers designed to promote skin healing and collagen development may be beneficial for your skin after treatment. Products containing hyaluronic acid aid in moisture retention, and vitamin C serums encourage antioxidant defense and skin lightening.

Between Vampire Facial treatments, adding retinoids or peptides can improve skin firmness and texture even further. These components increase collagen production and cell turnover, extending PRP's restorative benefits. Sunscreen with broad-spectrum SPF protection is essential to maintain the skin's tone and clarity after vampire facials and to stop UV-induced damage.

Furthermore, by sustaining skin suppleness and promoting continued collagen formation, growth factor-containing treatments can be used in conjunction with vampire facials. By encouraging cellular renewal and repair, these formulas strengthen the skin's natural defenses against outside stresses and the early indications of aging.

Speaking with a skincare expert can help you choose products that will work best for your skin type and post-vampire Facial treatment objectives. To guarantee long-term skin health and maximize treatment results, they might suggest customized skincare regimens. You may maintain the results of Vampire Facials and eventually attain radiant, youthful-looking skin by incorporating potent skincare products into your everyday routine.

FAQS: WHAT OTHER TREATMENTS CAN I GET IN ADDITION TO A VAMPIRE FACIAL?

Depending on your skincare objectives and treatment plan, combining a vampire facial with other skincare procedures can often be useful. Combining vampire facials with microneedling sessions improves the effects of skin renewal and collagen formation. Fine wrinkles and acne scars can be effectively reduced and overall skin texture can be improved with this combination. Additionally, by addressing certain issues like sun damage, age spots, and uneven skin tone, combining Vampire Facials with chemical peels or laser treatments can improve skincare outcomes even more.

To find the best combination therapies for your skin type and desired results, it's imperative to speak with a licensed skincare specialist. Experts can design a customized course of treatment that optimizes effectiveness and reduces possible negative effects. To attain the best possible rejuvenation and long-term skin health, they will also monitor how your skin responds to the combination of treatments and modify the procedures as necessary.

Under the supervision of a professional, combining Vampire Facials with complementary treatments can expedite skin renewal and address several skincare issues at once.

CHAPTER ELEVEN
COMMON QUESTIONS AND EXTENSIVE ANSWERS
RESOLVING PAIN AND UNEASE

A vampire facial includes the use of platelet-rich plasma (PRP) and microneedling, both of which can be uncomfortable to differing degrees. PRP can fully permeate the skin since the technique involves puncturing the skin with small needles, which stimulate the synthesis of collagen. Even though numbing cream is usually used beforehand to reduce pain, some people may still feel a little uncomfortable or like they're being slightly pinched or pricked. For the majority of people, this feeling is controllable and rapidly goes away after treatment.

Practitioners make sure the numbing lotion covers the treatment region completely to effectively relieve any discomfort during the vampire facial. They might also modify the microneedling depth based on each patient's unique sensitivity threshold.

It is recommended that patients be candid with their provider on any discomfort they may have throughout the process since it is frequently possible to improve comfort levels without sacrificing the outcome. While some people may experience some discomfort during the Vampire Facial, most people believe that the advantages outweigh any short-term discomfort.

CONTROLLING RESULTS-RELATED EXPECTATIONS

When thinking about getting a vampire facial, it's important to know that results can vary based on specific skin types and issues. Through the promotion of skin regeneration and stimulation of collagen formation, the treatment seeks to improve skin tone, texture, and overall look. Although many patients experience changes in skin texture and radiance right away after the first session, the best effects usually show up over a few weeks as collagen continues to rebuild.

Patients must be aware that although Vampire Facials might produce dramatic benefits, it may take several sessions spaced several weeks apart to have the best effects.

Professionals frequently offer advice on a customized treatment plan depending on the aims and concerns of each patient's skin. Patients can more fully enjoy the transforming advantages of the Vampire Facial by having reasonable expectations and being aware of the progressive nature of collagen stimulation techniques.

POSSIBLE HAZARDS AND SAFETY ISSUES

The vampire facial is usually thought to be safe, but like any cosmetic operation, there are certain hazards and things to keep in mind. The main dangers are mild bruising, swelling, and transient redness at the treatment site, which usually goes away in a few days. To reduce the danger of infection, equipment must be properly sterilized and hygiene precautions must be followed.

To guarantee that the proper measures are taken, patients with sensitive skin or a history of skin disorders should disclose these to their providers.

More serious side effects, like PRP allergies or excessive bleeding at the microneedling sites, can sporadically happen. When sterile methods are used and the procedure is carried out by a skilled practitioner, these situations are rare. To promote healing and reduce hazards, patients are urged to carefully adhere to post-care instructions, which may include limiting sun exposure and utilizing skincare products that are suggested.

LONG-TERM ADVANTAGES AND UPKEEP

The Vampire Facial's long-term advantages include smoother, more youthful-looking skin, fewer wrinkles and fine lines, and increased skin renewal. Through the promotion of natural healing processes and stimulation of collagen formation, the treatment can help preserve the appearance of youthful skin over time.

Practitioners frequently advise a course of treatments followed by sporadic maintenance sessions to maximize and prolong effects.

The benefits of a regular skincare regimen, such as hydrating, protecting against the sun, and mild washing, are enhanced by the vampire facial. To support skin health and maximize the long-term effects of treatment, patients are recommended to follow healthy lifestyle practices like drinking plenty of water, eating a balanced diet high in antioxidants, and quitting smoking. Through the implementation of these techniques, people can maintain and improve the outcomes of the Vampire Facial for a longer duration.

FAQS: HOW DO I PROCEED IF I ENCOUNTER UNANTICIPATED SIDE EFFECTS?

After receiving a vampire facial, it's critical to get in touch with your healthcare professional right away if you have any unexpected adverse effects.

While mild bruising, swelling, or redness is normal and normally goes away on its own, prolonged pain, severe discomfort, or any indications of infection should be reported right once. To reduce discomfort and encourage healing, providers may suggest topical treatments or prescription drugs. They can also provide advice on how to manage symptoms.

Patients should carefully adhere to post-care instructions, which usually involve avoiding harsh skincare products, prolonged sun exposure, and physically demanding activities that may aggravate side effects. As instructed, keep the treated area clean and moisturized to help improve skin healing and lessen discomfort. Above all, keeping lines of communication open with your doctor guarantees prompt attention and customized treatment, which can help you deal with unforeseen side effects and protect the health of your skin after treatment.

www.ingramcontent.com/pod-product-compliance
Lightning Source LLC
Chambersburg PA
CBHW061251250726

48653CB00002B/610